Tried and Tested Medicinal Herbs
by Dr. Carol Batey-Prunty

Cover by John Prunty
Edited by Katie Shea

March 2018

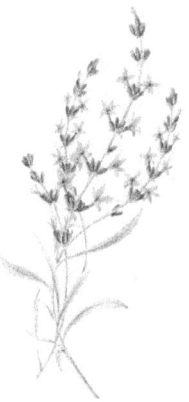

My Dear,

I designed this little booklet to provide easy reading for you. I began allowing plants to speak directly to my soul over thirty-nine years ago. I learned to listen to them with my inner ear and to use my intuition to learn from them. I encourage you to do the same! May you always be in harmony with all plants, herbs, flowers, bees, and trees. This peaceful harmony is imperative for you to cultivate a healthy mind, body, and spirit.

Green Blessings,
Carol

For my supportive husband, John E. Prunty

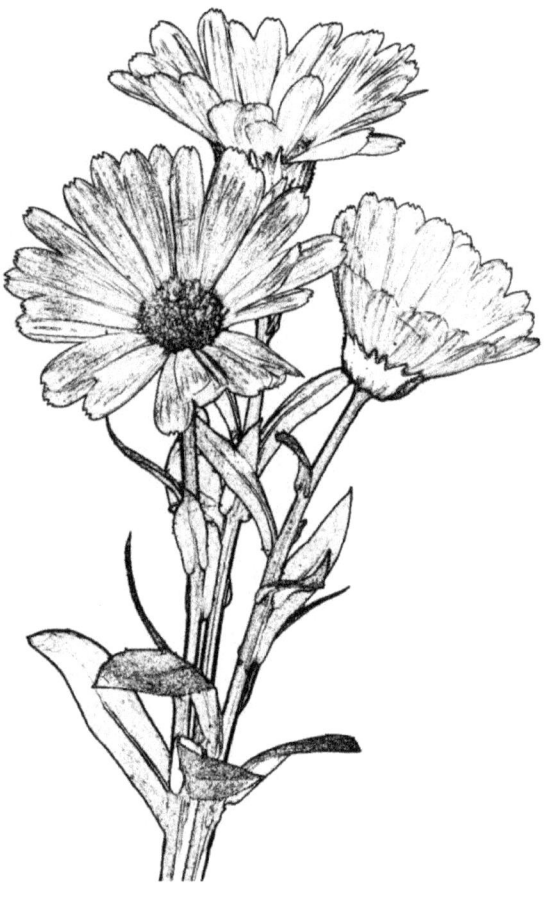

Table of Contents

Plants Speak: Dandelion (*Taraxacum officinale*) 1

Plants Speak: Yarrow (*Achillea millefolium*) 4

Plants Speak: Calendula (*Calendula officinalis*) 6

Plants Speak: Comfrey (*Symphytum officinale*) 8

Plants Speak: Common Thyme (*Thymus vulgaris*) 10

Plants Speak: Solomon's Seal 12

Plants Speak: Common Plantain (*Plantago major*) 14

Plants Speak: Mullein (*Verbascum thapsus*) 17

Plants Speak: Rosemary (*Rosmarinus officinalis*) 19

Plants Speak: Meadowsweet (*Filipendula ulmaria*) 21

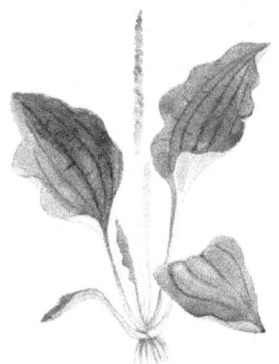

Carol's Beginnings

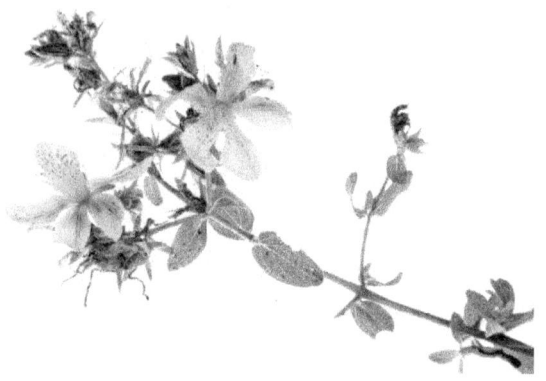

As a young child, I was sensitive to people and my surroundings. I could pick up other people's thoughts. I intuitively knew if they were sick, happy, or sad. Often, I would hear footsteps within the house when no one else did. Later, I started to see spirits of people who were not alive anymore. Being a small child, I thought I was crazy. I didn't have any adults that I could confide in, so I decided to keep my mouth shut!

My mother often told me that I had Indian blood just like my father, whom I never lived with or knew! My father was half Cherokee and African American. When I became an adult, I went to my father's family to find out more about his heritage, because he was deceased. I found out that I was just like him. His family told me about my grandma, Anna, who was Cherokee. Anna would dig up Dandelion roots daily and boil them in water, adding honey to it for the family to drink. She completed this action every morning. As a result, her family was rarely sick.

Learning about my family brought me closer to my father and sparked my desire to learn more about medicinal plants. In 1982, I started to investigate the healing powers of the herbal plants that I had in my backyard. Around this time, I became sick. After seeking proper medical attention, I still wasn't feeling better. This prompted me to seek a solution outside of conventional Western medicine. I became connected with an underground herbal group in Nashville, Tennessee. This "green-team" taught me about herbs and their healing power. As I began working with herbs and their healing properties, I began to notice what worked for me and what didn't. My ex-husband and I had six children. I used herbs to help my children with common ailments. I had a lot of success, but I learned through trial and error. Through experience, I discovered that, if I listened closely enough, the plants would speak to me. I know the same can be true for you with practice!

Years later, I went to massage school where I was introduced to essential oils. In 1997, I took herbal classes in Atlanta with Patricia Kyritsi Howell. It was at this workshop that I first learned to make skin-care salves. After this workshop, I attended Patricia's school, and I took herbal preparation classes in my hometown, Red Boiling Springs, Tennessee. By this time, I had graduated from taking herbs internally and began applying them externally! The next year, I went to skin-care school. I enjoyed creating herbal products for the whole body and exploring the different ways that herbs may be used internally and externally.

I am a firm believer that plants speak to us, and it is our job to listen to them. For example, Dandelion (*Taraxacum officinale*) loves to share that she is a faithful weed that can heal many things within the body. She speaks to us within the sacred spaces of kitchens, creams, wines, jellies, salads, incense and herbal medicines. Thinking Dandelion is just a troublesome weed, most people want to pluck her out of their yards. It is the purpose of this book to acquaint you with Dandelion and other plants and to help you begin listening to their healing wisdom.

It is likely that you already have extensive experience with medicinal plants! Common medicinal plants are used as spices and herbs in cooking. Likewise, flower and vegetable gardens are brimming with medicinal opportunities.

Here is a small testament of tried and tested herbal knowledge and how to make herbal products from plants that I grow in my own backyard herbal garden. I encourage you to try these techniques for yourself. Be sure to listen closely to the wisdom of the plants! Remember to always research plants before using them. **Please note, the information in this book is not a substitute for professional medical care. You should always consult your physician before using any herbs internally or externally.**

Green Blessings,
Carol

Plants Speak: Dandelion (*Taraxacum officinale*)

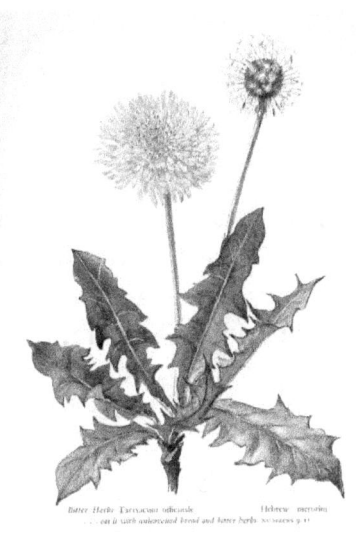

Hi! My name is Dandelion, officially known as *Taraxacum officinal*. A 15th-century surgeon gave me my name when he looked at my leaf and thought, "it's shaped like a lion tooth." People who want beautiful yards, without weeds, use herbicide or pesticides on me! I wish they were aware that I am a plant with extraordinary healing properties! I am known to live, grow, and thrive all over the world. I came to the Americas by way of the Mayflower ship. From there, my hearty roots set into soil across Canada, California, and Mexico. My strong roots have been used since the 10th century. In Ancient Rome and Arab countries, doctors recommended my leaves to be used as a diuretic. Coffee drinkers loved drinking herbal, caffeine-free tea made from my edible roots.

I have multiple uses, and I can heal many ailments in the body. I can assist digestion. I am a natural diuretic and rich in potassium. Do you have a sluggish liver, gallbladder, or intestines? Try my dandelion root tea to eliminate toxins and provide relief from arthritis and gout. You can make a decoction by boiling my deep brown roots in hot water.

When making a tincture, you may use fresh or dried herbs. I suggest you use fresh or dried flowers, leaves, seeds, or stems. Always use clean herbs. You may chop or grind them in a spice grinder. Beginning in January through the end of March, Carol drinks my tincture (in water) and my tea three up to times a day. I spoke to her and she listened.

Every part of me may be eaten. My fresh flowers may be added to any salad. Do you cook greens? Add some fresh dandelions to your next batch of fried or steamed vegetables. You may juice my leaves for an added boost of Vitamin A, B, C, and D.

Harvest me anytime during the growing season. Make sure that I have not been sprayed and do not harvest me from a roadside. When harvesting, please remember to leave some of me behind to continue to grow. Always remember to give thanks to me and the Creator of all things!

To make Dandelion Root Tea: Bring water to a boil and turn off the burner. Add dandelion seeds, berries, flowers, roots, stems and leaves. Cover and steep for 15 minutes or more. Strain out the herbal compound inside the decoction and enjoy your tea! Optional: Add honey to taste.

To make a Dandelion Tincture: Get a clean jar. Pack chopped herbs and top with alcohol. Use 90 proof or more pure grain alcohol or vodka. Date and label the jar. After six weeks, strain through a cheesecloth and wring the cheesecloth with clean hands. Put 3 eye droppers of this tincture in tea or water to drink up to three times a day.

To make a Dandelion Jelly: Make a strong infusion of dandelion, using all parts of the plant. An infusion is made with hot water. Let the dandelion sit in the water for one day. Next, make Dandelion Jelly by using 2 cups of strong infusion, ½ cup of cider vinegar, 2 ½ cups of honey. Then, add 3 oz. of fruit pectin to the liquid and place on the stove. Bring the liquid to a boil. Put into a clean sterilized jar. You may put into the refrigerator for later use on toast.

Plants Speak: Yarrow (*Achillea millefolium*)

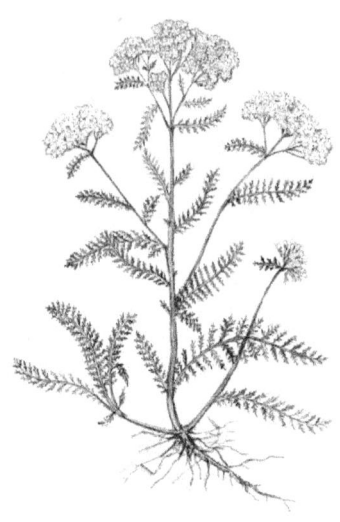

At one time, I was known to heal almost everything on the planet! I am still known for my magnificent powers. My plant is an astringent, and my very own oils are an antiseptic. Does your blood need to be cleansed? My leaves contain chlorophyll, which will cleanse your blood. When the Greeks went to war, they used my magical plant to cleanse and stop bleeding in their feet and tendons—their "Achilles!"

You may crush my fresh leaves and apply them directly to sprains or other inflamed areas of the body. This will start the healing process, stopping inflammation and bleeding. I am a perfect staple for any first aid kit. I can help nose bleeds, infections, colds, flu, and fever. I can also assist diuretic, lung, digestive, and rheumatic issues. Father Kneipp of Germany thought so much of me, he wanted people to juice me for the healing of tumors, psoriasis, and the treatment of really bad wounds. Every part of my plant may be used to treat issues in the body.

In addition to treating the body, I am used as dye to color items yellow, in cosmetics, and to make herbal wine and beer.

If you have a problem with bugs in the spring, summer or fall, you may add me to bug repellent for additional benefits. Hikers, climbers and runners, who travel through woods, need me in their pocket for "first aid." When Carol makes bug repellent for her customers, she uses my fresh or dried flowers in her oils. She makes a bug repellent lotion bar with beeswax and a bug repellent spray with water, vodka, and added plants.

To make Yarrow Face Wash for Blackheads: Soak 2 tbsp. of chopped yarrow (fresh or dried) in 2 oz. cold milk. Let sit overnight. The next day, strain out the herb. Use as face wash. Warm before use on your face if you desire. You may also drink this daily for best results.

Plants Speak: Calendula (*Calendula officinalis*)

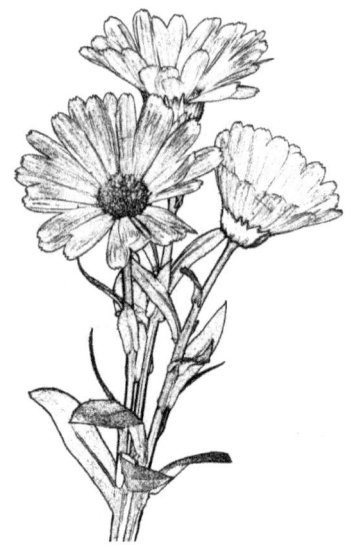

I have been called a ray of sunshine because of my bright yellowish-gold color. Although I don't grow back every year, my flower petals drop into soil, enabling more growth. Put me into the sun to grow, and I will! Harvest me once my petals open. The Romans loved my plants and named me in honor of my ability to bloom on the first of every month in warm weather! One of my other names is "Pot of Marigold" because of my yellow color and the way my petals enrich the flavor of soups. This is not to be confused with the marigold flower plants, which are edible but have no healing properties.

I have healing properties within my whole flower and green stems. I am nutritiously packed with antioxidants, lutein, beta-carotene, and Vitamin A. Try me in a garden salad or mixed into rice. My yellow color will come into the rice, giving you a visual sense of my healing presence.

You are probably wondering about my healing abilities. I stimulate the healing of chronic fungal infections, ringworm, mouth disorders, muscle spasms, and yeast infections. I am particularly good at healing skin interruptions and wounds. My oil makes the best massage oils and salves and will make your skin soft. Carol uses me in almost all of her herbal skin-care creations.

To make Calendula Oil: Pick calendula flowers early in the morning. Once the petals have opened, you may put the flowers into a 16 oz. jar. Fill to the top. Add Olive Oil or Almond Oil. Cover with a lid and put in the sun for two weeks. Shake the jar every day. After two weeks, strain with a cheesecloth. Place the antiseptic oil in a jar or bottle for later use.

Plants Speak: Comfrey (*Symphytum officinale*)

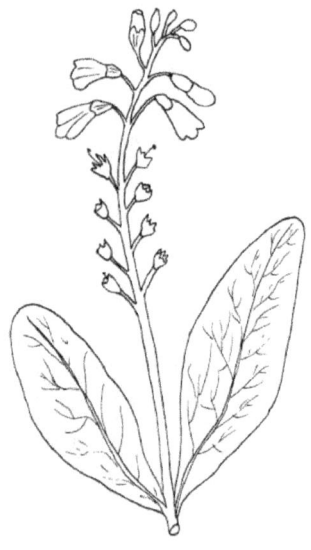

I am excellent medicine for other plant crops and for you! Many people use me to mulch over other plants. Once I start growing in your yard, it is hard to kill me. I give plants potassium and other nutrients. However, I do have a high amount of carcinogenic properties, so please do not take me by mouth.

Use my tincture or cream on your skin, and you will heal quickly. I heal pulled muscles, fractures, burns, and bruises. I can also stop a cut from bleeding! The American Indians named me "knit bones," because I facilitate fractured bones during the healing process. If you use me daily, my oils can rebuild your cells.

To make a Comfrey Salve: Pick comfrey early in the morning and dry off. Next, shred the leaves into a clean 8 oz. jar. Fill the jar to the top with flowers and pour Olive Oil over them. Put in a dark place for three weeks. After three weeks, strain with a cheesecloth. In a double boiler on low heat, add 2 oz. of beeswax for melting. Then, add 2 cups of comfrey oil. Watch the beeswax melt. Carol loves to add lavender essential oil and peppermint oil to soothe and heal bones and muscles.

Plants Speak: Common Thyme (*Thymus vulgaris*)

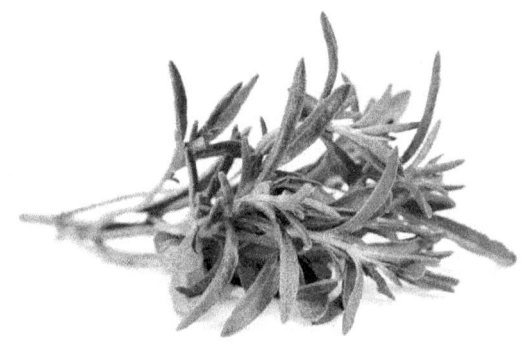

I am a little seed that produces a lot of shrubby plants. I am a powerful antiseptic. I have many different types, and I grow back each year. I like being planted near rocks, in full sun, and with little water. Harvest every part of my herb from early summer through early fall. I come from Europe and the northern shores of the Mediterranean. In the temples of Greece, my plant was burned as incense and used as perfume.

I am excellent to cook with and to eat. You may add me to olives, soups and stews, chicken, fish, dressings, and cheese.

In World War II, I was burned with rosemary (my cousin) in hospitals. I was used to purify illnesses in the hospital rooms. My oil contains thymol. Thymol disinfects all bacteria from surfaces. You may use me to clean your office or home.

I can help many issues that occur in the body, including muscle spasms, eczema, pleurisy, whooping cough, skin issues, sore throats, and ulcers. I am a go-to herb. Your lungs will call my name! You may put me into a syrup, and I will help! I also can assist children, who have pinworms within their bodies. **Do not give this syrup to children under 2 years old.**

To make Thyme Syrup: Pack about ¾ cup fresh and dried thyme in a clean 8 oz. jar. Fill jar with about ¼ cup lemon rind (organic if possible) and top with honey (use pure honey for the thyme syrup if possible). Label and date.

Thyme syrup should last for six months. You may give one tablespoon of thyme syrup to a child to expel worms and to assist coughs. This syrup can be added to a cup of herbal tea for additional medicinal benefits.

To make Herbal Thyme Salt: Dry thyme in an oven at 150 degrees on parchment paper and until the herb is completely dried. Put the dried herb into a food processor. Measure out 1 cup and add to this mixture to ½ cup sea salt. Blend both together in a food processor. Store in a jar for later use.

Plants Speak: Solomon's Seal
(*Polygonatum multiflorum*)

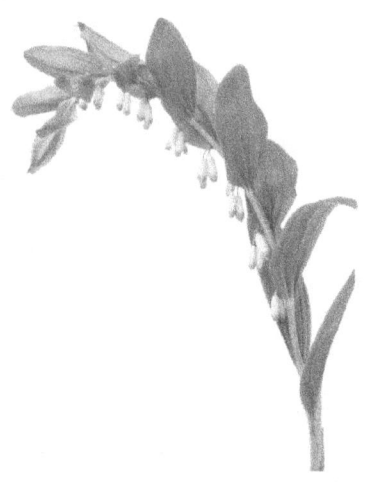

Carol discovered my roots last year at the annual Folk Medicine Festival in Red Boiling Springs, Tennessee. She her husband were vendors this festival. Carol found me at another vendor's booth and, after much research, began to add me to her repertoire of go-to herbs.

I grow below the ground. In the fall, my roots can be harvested. My leaves are so beautiful, making a bell-shape at the top with a blueish flower fruit blooming outward. My stem is a *rhizome*, which means that it grows horizontally underground and then puts out shoots that go sideways!

I act like a steroid, and I have a lot of vitamin A! I can be traced back to 1st century China. The American Indians of Maine, the Penobscot, used me to help treat gonorrhea. The North American Indians used my healing properties daily to aid the healing of muscles, tendons, inflammation, torn cartilage, and bones. I love to heal shoulder and neck issues! My roots work better when they are combined with other similar herbs, such as boneset.

Comfrey and boneset work in partnership with me to repair bone fractures. You may make an oil, tincture, or salve with our three ingredients. I can be applied to heal osteoarthritis and injuries. My oil should be in every emergency kit.

To make Solomon's Seal Oil (with Comfrey and Boneset): Using fresh or dried herbs, put all three herbs into a clean jar and top with Almond Oil. If the weather is above 70 degrees Fahrenheit, put the jar outside. Keep in the sun to prep for seven days. Shake the jar daily. After seven days, strain the herbs using a cheesecloth and place the oil into a jar for later use.
Optional: Add 30 drops of peppermint essential oil.

Plants Speak: Common Plantain (*Plantago major*)

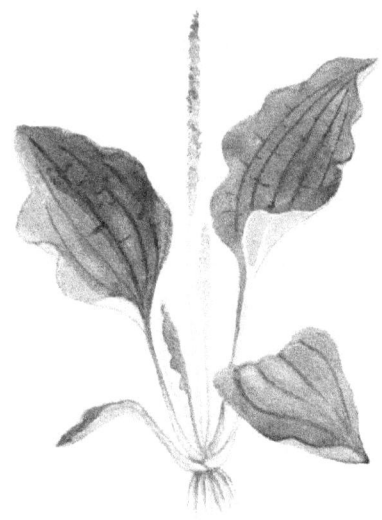

The English settlers brought me to the Americas and introduced me to the American Indians, who began calling me way-bread. However, most of you call me common plantain. I am a healing herb with broad oval-shaped leaves. I love growing in yards, playgrounds, meadows, and pathways. I am both a medicinal plant and a food crop. Home-owners and gardeners tend to get rid of me, but I am extremely useful in healing various conditions.

I have many uses. My leaves contain aucubin, which helps heal sore throats and removes uric acid from toes when gout is present. Many people use me for indigestion and diarrhea. My seeds can be turned into an herbal laxative. I can draw toxins out of the body. You may use me for healing your blood. Cleansing blood is what I do best!

I am edible and taste great in salad. I contain vitamin A, which is necessary for healthy eyes, healing skin eruptions, and a healthy liver. Believe it or not, I contain more vitamin A than carrots! You may drink me in an herbal tea made from fresh or dried leaves. Carol loves to juice me or add my fresh leaves, with other vegetables, to her smoothies.

My fresh leaves are best used on the skin in a poultice. A poultice is made by combining chopped, fresh herbs with hot boiling water.

Carol uses my leaves in almost everything she makes. She adds me to her herbal bug repellent formula. I add an astringent action to bug repellent and any other salve that is made with me. I also stop the sting and relieve the itchiness and redness of bug bites. I should advise you to put my salve in your first aid kit.

To make a Plantain Poultice: Pick my herb from an unsprayed yard. Wash the leaves in water and dry them off. Chop up the leaves in a food processor. Then, apply a small amount of hot water to the leaves. After 2-3 minutes apply to wounds, stings, sores, or burns. Wrap with gauze to hold my herbal poultice in place.

To make a Plantain Salve: Use a clean 2 oz. jar. Pick about 2 oz. of plantain from the yard. In a double boiler, put me in Olive Oil on low for two hours. (The boiler should have about 3 cups of water in it.) Strain my herbs out of the pan. Next, put 1 oz. beeswax in a double boiler, still on low, and add my oil to melt the beeswax. Pour the oil into a cream jar. Label and date! (Note: you may substitute Olive Oil with Almond or Coconut Oil.)

Plants Speak: Mullein (*Verbascum thapsus*)

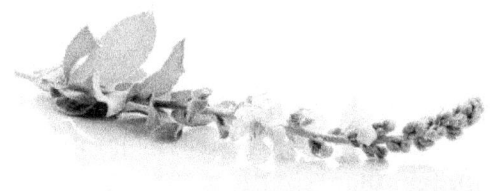

I am a wayside herbal weed that often grows in rocks along the freeway. While driving, you may see my yellow, spikey flowers. I did not grow the first year Carol planted me in her garden, but I grew very well the second year. I do not need any special care. Every part of my spikey plant may be used to heal your body. Do you have eye problems, toothaches, earaches, asthma, or a cough? I can even fight tuberculosis! Come straight to me, and I will help you heal.

Many herbalists have found me to be an antispasmodic, which means that I can relax muscle spasms. The American Indians rolled my large, hairy leaves and smoked me, along with other herbs, for asthma. Carol drinks me with her other herbs three times a day for her glandular health. You may make a poultice out of my leaves to use for swelling, insect bites, and more. You may add my dried or fresh leaves and flowers to your bath water to soothe rheumatic pains. Carol makes her own Elderberry cough syrup and adds me to her mixture for added protection against a cough. When Carol has an earache, my oil is able to move the fluid in her ears. When Carol's joints ache, she rubs my oil into her muscles. This helps ease the pain for a while!

I suggest you have me on hand in your medicine chest and first aid kit!

To make Mullein Ear Oil: Put 1quart Olive Oil into a clean jar. Add 10 garlic cloves to the jar and ½ cup fresh or dried mullein plant. In the summer, let the jar sit in a sunny space outside to infuse for two weeks. Strain the herb and store the oil in brown glass in your medicine chest.

To use: Fill an eye dropper and place into your ears. Repeat until your ear is full. Place a cotton ball over your ear to soak up excess oil.

To make Mullein Tea: Put 1 tbsp. mullein in 1 cup boiling water. Strain to drink.

Plants Speak: Rosemary (*Rosmarinus officinalis*)

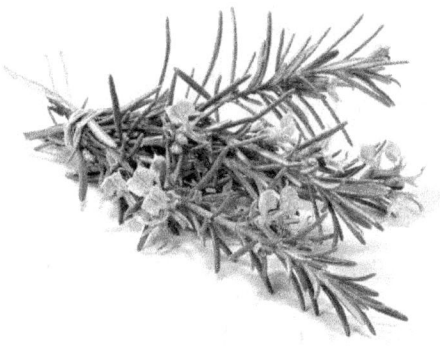

Many people love me! I am a common herb in many foods. My essential oil is often used in diffusers, sprays, and muscle soaks. What most people don't know is that they can enhance their memory and cognition just by smelling my leaves and flowers! In the past, students have tied a ring of my flowers and leaves around their heads to improve attention and memory retention. I am a shrub with fragrant flowers that hails from near the Mediterranean. I am often referred to as "dew of the sea." If I am protected with hay or have burlap bags over me, I can grow in cold weather.

I can help elderly people by stimulating them in body, mind, and spirit. I am an astringent in nature. Therefore, I can reduce germs in a house, office, or car! Spray my essential oils to purify your environment and improve cognition! Ancient Egyptians, Romans, and Greeks found me to be sacred in their temples and homes. I assist the healthy functioning of the bowels, stomach, and spleen. Aerial parts, which are all parts of my woody leaves, are used to improve circulation. **Do not use me if you have epilepsy or pregnant.**

Carol makes and drinks 2 quarts of an herbal blend of tea daily. Sometimes, Carol adds 4 eye droppers of my tincture to her tea. You may make a tincture from my leaves by following the recipe for the dandelion tincture on page 3. Simply substitute dandelions with rosemary leaves. Carol trusts that I will help her muscles move in her body, and she uses me for gastric disturbances. My leaves help with bile production in the liver. **Be sure to consult your physician before trying this or any other method in this booklet.**

I also can calm your nerves, lower blood pressure, and work on pest control. Carol adds me to her bug repellent lotion bar that has over thirty herbs and spices and ten essential oils

I am excellent in hair and on skin! I can help dry, brittle hair and dandruff by stimulating the nerves and roots.

To make the Rosemary Hair Rejuvenator: Put dry or fresh rosemary leaves in a clean 8 oz. jar. Top with witch hazel and 10 drops of pure organic rosemary essential oil from a health food store. Leave for about two days in the sun and then strain the leaves. Apply to your scalp and wet or dry hair. Put a shower cap on your hair for one hour. After an hour, rinse your hair in water.

Plants Speak: Meadowsweet (*Filipendula ulmaria*)

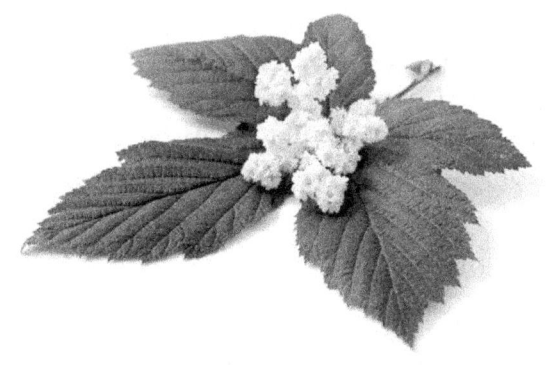

I am the "Queen of the Meadow." Build a strong relationship with me, and I will support your healing. My leaves and flowers have been used throughout Europe. My flowers are used for a honey wine called mead. Mead is a wine that is fermented with water, yeast and, honey. Other plants, like dandelion, chamomile, and more, can be used to make mead.

In 1853, an Italian professor discovered my healing abilities. One of my compounds is salicylic. In 1899, the Bayer company, created Bayer Aspirin from my salicylic compound. White Willow Bark (my cousin) also contains salicylic and was used by Bayer to create aspirin.

My actions are cooling, and I can remove stagnant energy from one's body. I am a natural antacid, and I assist with stomach issues, ulcers, reflux, digestion problems, and Irritable Bowel Syndrome. My leaves and flowers neutralize the acid in the stomach. I am an anti-inflammatory, and I can move bones and muscle. I love to help small children with headaches and colic.

When Carol first learned about me, she began drinking me along with her tea infusion 8 herbs daily for rheumatic problems. She has been enlightened to my wonderful sacred healing of gastritis and indigestion. As she develops a long-lasting relationship with me and allows my vibrations to carry into her heart and soul, she is awakening to my helpfulness.

To Make Carol's 8 Herb Tea: Gather eight herbs (dandelion, nettles, meadowsweet, ginkgo, plantain, calendula, mint, and *comfrey). Put 1 tsp. of each herb into a 1-quart jar. Fill the jar up with hot boiling water and cover. Wait one hour before straining the herbs. After one hour, your tea is ready to be consumed. Carol likes to set her intention for why she is drinking the tea and gives thanks to each herb. (You may add 4 eye droppers of rosemary tincture to the tea if you would like for added medicinal benefits.)
*Carol drinks this blend with comfrey. Drink at your own risk, keeping in mind comfrey is high in carcinogenic properties.

We are now at the end of this little booklet. Thank you for reading about s plants that grow in Carol's herbal backyard garden. We love our home, and we welcome you to come visit us!

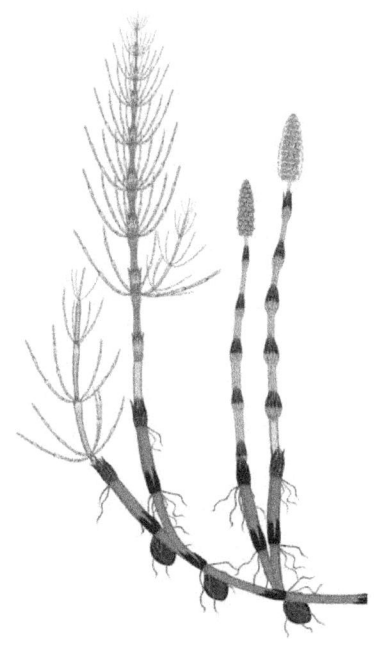

You can grow aromatic herbal medicine outside in your backyard.

www.ingramcontent.com/pod-product-compliance
Lightning Source LLC
Chambersburg PA
CBHW071000220526
45471CB00007B/3109